It's All About Love

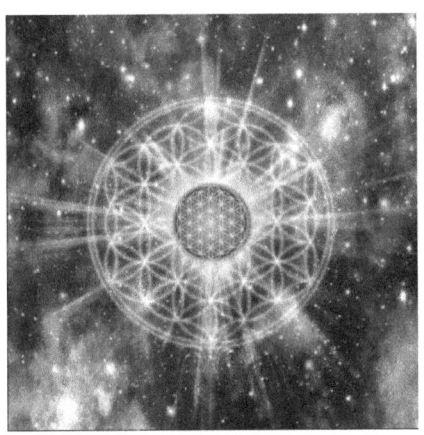

Sandra Munro

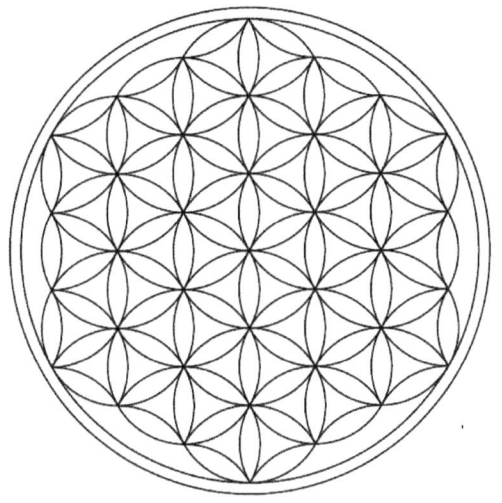

It's All

About Love

Acknowledgement

There are so many people in my life who have provided inspiration on the path; my beautiful husband, two daughters and sweet grandchildren, my beloved teacher Gurumayi, as well as my friends Kay and Norma who gently took me by the hand and led me out of the shadows from time to time. Our interaction together on this journey has found me dipping into the well of unconditional love again and again until eventually, I became **THAT**.

ABOUT THE AUTHOR

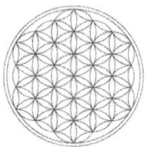

Sandra has worked in many fields including the law, television, theatre, the corporate world, interior design, retailing, real estate and property development. Her most recent occupation was teaching, where she worked with young children for more than twenty years.

In 1989 she was diagnosed with cancer. The disease was not only fast-moving but life-threatening, yet despite a prediction of only a few weeks to live and through the deep exploration of what was thought of at the time as alternate therapy, she experienced a phenomenon explained by the medical profession as 'a spontaneous remission'.

Once recovered, her search for the meaning of life began in earnest and as her journey unfolded she began to develop a philosophy that by taking a series of simple steps, it was not only possible to *change* the direction of your life, but empower yourself to embrace *whatever* comes your way in a spirit of joy and adventure.

Sandra insists that she is just a messenger and her role is to inspire others to embrace their own mastery.

Married for more than forty-six years she has two grown daughters and five grandchildren and currently lives on the beautiful south coast of New South Wales, Australia where she finds much inspiration for her writing.

From the seed of Truth comes purity and from the words of the Master

'Consider the lilies of the field'; an indication of the white Light emerging from the

depths of darkness and when Light is obtained the gold appears....clumps of these

creations of our Heavenly Father indicate the emerging of the buds unfolding to be

revealed in all their beauty.

PROLOGUE

This is a story about my personal journey from darkness into the light. It began when I was challenged with a fast-moving form of Leukemia and found me enmeshed in a world in where I totally believed that the odds were stacked against me. From this dark place I was shown a chink of light; a way out of my predicament and I knew that if I decided to follow this path, incredibly and perhaps miraculously, it would lead me to its source and I could step up and claim the light as my own.

INDEX

Chapter One

Little Hiccups

Remember, it is not the thing believed in,

but the belief in your own mind

that brings about the results.

The Power of Your Subconscious Mind – Joseph Murphy

As I gently put the groceries down on the bench and removed my hand from the gaping hole in the bottom of the paper bag, I thought that being environmentally aware was one thing but sometimes the alternatives left a lot to be desired. I sighed to myself, cocking one ear to the ruckus going on upstairs between my two daughters who were arguing over something I couldn't quite decipher.

I rubbed my temples which were tight from the drive home in the traffic and went outside again to gather the remainder of my shopping from the car boot. As I slowly unpacked the groceries, absentmindedly putting them in the fridge, I surveyed the choices for dinner, mentally calculating how their preparation fitted with my energy levels, which had been down of late.

Once this task was done I hurried upstairs and greeted the girls who hardly took a breath from their debate, and popped into the bathroom for a moment where I caught my reflection in the mirror and as I gazed at the lumps which filled out my neck on one side, I wondered if they were really swollen glands from a recent Flu. They didn't seem to change or go down much, even though the Flu symptoms had disappeared long ago. Aside from this I felt well but tiered, as life always seemed so busy these days.

The latch on the front door clicked shut and I realized that my husband was home so I rushed downstairs to greet him and put on the tea. Lately I never knew what mood he would be in. His job was stressful and sometimes he just needed to let off steam when he came home, so I steeled myself in case this was one of those days. To my relief he seemed happy but absent-minded, going into the lounge room to switch on the television. He enjoyed watching the evening news and this was a ritual which never varied. I bustled about in the kitchen preparing the meal and felt slightly put out that he hadn't given me his usual "hello" peck on the cheek. Later as I lay in bed, my fingers strayed to the lumps on my neck once more and I wondered, probably for the hundredth time, when they would go away.

I had been a teacher for many years and was beginning to find my profession more and more challenging and was constantly trying to think of an alternate way to earn my living when an idea, which had been percolating in my mind for quite a while, began to surface. I had always enjoyed decorating my home and as my husband and I had bought and sold many properties over the years, I knew that the part which I enjoyed most about this venture was having a fresh canvas to decorate each time. With this in mind, I began to explore the possibility of opening a shop where I could capitalize on these ideas.

No sooner had I given this concept my attention when my mind began to explode with possibilities. I discussed it with my husband over dinner and interestingly, he was very keen to finance it but there was one stipulation; he insisted I go into business with my sister-in-law. As a businessman, he could see the practicality of this. Retailing could be a tiring and exasperating profession and having had his own business when he was younger and knowing the pitfalls of going it alone, felt that a partnership was the ideal way to go.

I could feel my opposition to this scheme begin to engulf me. This was my adventure and I was not sure how my sister-in-law would fit into the picture and although we got on well, we were both strong women. While I knew the idea might appeal to her, I was not sure how it would work out. My husband was adamant however; if I wanted the shop, my sister-in-law had to be part of the deal.

I discovered a little shop across the road from the local railway station which seemed the ideal choice. There were plenty of people passing by and the stock I planned to display was quite different to anything being offered in the immediate vicinity. It seemed too good an opportunity to pass up and after trying one more time to convince my husband that I could do this alone, his firm stance sent me off in the direction of my sister-in-laws's house to discuss the project. As I walked the short distance, I wondered yet again if I was doing the right thing.

My sister-in-law was delighted with the idea and told me she had always wanted to work in retail and as we began to attend trade fairs to seek out the kind of stock I wanted to provide, I found that for the most part, our taste in merchandise was pretty similar, which was a plus. The rent on the small shop was reasonable and things seemed to be going well; a fresh coat of paint, some carpet and attractive window décor and we were ready to go.

I soon became enmeshed in the creative stimulation of the lead-up to the opening of the business. There was a lot to do and while we were busy with the selection and ordering of stock, we kept the window covered with brown paper to keep the prying eyes of the public away; at least until opening time.

My tiredness had intensified but I had convinced myself that it was largely due to the demands which still needed to be seen to before the opening date. We were attending to some pre-opening tasks, when my sister-in-law asked me to pass something up from the box below and as I reached down to retrieve it, the room began to spin and I fainted.

When I opened my eyes, my sister-in-law was standing over me with a concerned look on her face. "Are you alright? You gave me such a fright," she said. I sat up slowly, rubbing the back of my head, which had struck the floor when I went down.

"I guess it is just tiredness. I have really been lacking in energy lately."

"I think you should go to the doctor and have it checked out", my sister-in-law said, her face betraying the thoughts that were going through her head at that moment; with only days to go before the opening, perhaps she was wondering if this was a foretaste of things to come.

Chapter Two

News

Your treasure house is within you.

Look within for the answers to your heart's desire

Anonymous

I knew there was a doctor's rooms just a few doors along from the shop and took myself up the stairs to the small surgery and sat down in the waiting room.

"What a strange thing," I thought to myself. "I have never fainted before. Hopefully, we will get to the bottom of it right now as there is still so much to do before we open."

Sitting there in that small waiting room, I mulled over the possibilities.

The doctor was quiet for what seemed like a long time and appeared very interested in the lumps on my neck.

"Just how long have you had them Mrs. Munro?"

I thought back to when they first became apparent. I had just had a bout of the Flu and had gone to my regular doctor to get something for it.

"I have had them for quite a while I think" I responded, "perhaps even a few months. I did speak to my doctor about them but he thought that they were swollen glands from the Flu".

The doctor wanted me to have a series of tests without delay as he suspected that the lumps might be something else. I felt my heart give a lurch.

"Something else, whatever could that be?" I wondered. I had been plagued with troubling health for the past three years, commencing with a viral eye infection which my husband had contracted in Bangkok and which was very contagious. His infection had cleared up after a few days but mine had caused me to have several weeks off work, as my eyes wouldn't heal and anybody who came into contact with me would manifest the same problem within a few days. The school principal very did not want me back at work until I was absolutely no longer contagious.

Once back at work, my energy levels seemed so low that the next cold developed into Pneumonia followed by Encephalitis which was an inflammation of the brain tissue. A long and severe bout of Depression had been the most recent development and it taken many months to pull myself back from this and now, here was another problem presenting itself just when we were about to go into a new business!

I felt frustrated by this new turn of events, however as I walked back down the stairs to the little shop to give my sister-in-law the news, I made light of it, explaining that I would need a few days to attend the hospital for some routine tests. Fortunately it did not mean we would have to postpone the opening, so at least that was a bonus.

The exploratory tests were mostly unpleasant and time-consuming and apart from the usual blood tests, I was asked to consume three tall glasses of a salty-tasting liquid. I was then injected with a substance which whizzed around my body at lightning speed (an exhilarating experience as it turned out) and as this foreign liquid pulsed throughout my system, the process was tracked; giving vital clues to the current state of my body.

The bone marrow extraction was next on the agenda and whilst I had refrained from obtaining details of this process in advance, the nurse soon informed me that it could be painful and encouraged me to feel free to express my discomfort as loudly as I wished; squeezing my hand tight in the process. Despite this warning, the actual extraction was not too daunting; in fact I had to ask when they had completed it as I hadn't felt much at all. The following day however, I awoke feeling as though I had been kicked by a mule and lay on the couch recuperating and feeling sorry for myself.

The last procedure was straight out of a hi-fi movie. After extracting some blood, it was irradiated with a nuclear substance and then re-injected into my body, which was then subjected to more scrutiny. These tiny irradiated particles highlighted any irregularities very efficiently and gave those examining the scans a very accurate picture of what was going on inside its most secret recesses.

Chapter Three

Strategy

In Divine Mind, there

is only perfection.

Nothing is Too Good to be True —John Randolph Price

There was one further test; a biopsy of the offending glands and the specialist who performed it had the kind of energy which portrayed him to be not only an expert in his field, but an impersonal one at that. Later, after the surgery which removed a Lymph node from my neck and one which necessitated cutting me across the throat almost from ear to ear, I spent the following week unable to eat as it hurt to move my jaw.

"At least I lost some weight", I joked to my sister-in-law, although it was painful to laugh.

I found myself sitting across from an Oncologist at the teaching hospital when the results came in. They revealed that the disease now had a name; Non-Hodgkin's Lymphoma, a-slow moving form of Cancer which was a member of the Leukemia family. This disease affected the Lymphatic system and one, according to the specialist, which was less-threatening than some of its cohorts. He told me that whilst the diagnosis was not good in that the disease would eventually prove fatal, in my particular case, it would only cut about seventeen or so years off my life expectancy. I looked at his face as he delivered this news.

"What was he talking about?" I am only forty-five, and as I began doing mental calculations in my mind, even with the best case scenario, this was going to dramatically affect my life.

I have always been stubborn, some would say that it was because I am a Taurean and others, who do not believe in such things, would just agree. I could dig my toes in and wait out the most insistent protagonist once I made up my mind about something and this news was making up my mind big time! As I looked at the kindly eyes of the doctor, I suspected that there was a lot he was not telling me. In the meantime, I gritted my teeth while silently shouting at him in my mind:

"That's what you think buster!" However out loud I said politely, "I suspect that you and I might be around long enough to laugh about this one day" and shook his hand before leaving the surgery.

Once back at the shop, I shared the news with my sister-in-law.

"It seems I am going to be around a long time yet." I said, smiling. Her expression did not give much clue to her feelings, but she put her arms around me and gave me a big hug and we began to unpack the remains of the stock which had arrived in my absence.

As there was no recommended treatment at this point in time and as I was feeling quite well, aside from the tiredness, my life went on in a fairly normal way; the only difference being that my husband was being strangely attentive and helpful. I began to bask in this extra consideration and wondered how long it would last.

Just before the diagnosis, we had decided to pull down our old house and build a new one and had moved into a little cottage across the road while all this took place. The cottage was very small and cramped, but I seemed to have been blessed with the special gift of making anywhere feel like home, a trait which had been honed over the years when we had been forced to relocate due to my husband's work.

My sister-in-law and her husband had also decided to move to a larger house just around the corner from where we currently lived. Their new home was spacious and set in lovely grounds right on the river, with a swimming pool placed invitingly in the garden. Their own house had been sold but it would be several weeks before the paperwork was completed and on receiving the news about my recent diagnosis, they suggested that perhaps my family might like to move into their new home to 'house sit' while waiting for our own house to be finished.

This seemed like a wonderful idea. I loved gardening and was looking forward to swimming in that lovely pool each morning. As most of our furniture was in storage, the move was accomplished quite quickly and we were settled within a few days. As I sat in the sun in the garden, I heaved a sigh of contentment and knew that these new surroundings could only help my situation as I always thrived in a beautiful environment.

The day after our move took place, we were in for a surprise. A removal truck pulled up out the front and my husband's mother walked down the path, followed by the removal men. Of course I knew that she would be living with my sister and brother-in-law eventually, after all they had bought the house together, but it never occurred to me that it would happen several weeks ahead of schedule.

Some years before, I had lived with my mother-in-law and although she was usually a lovely woman, caring and kind to the children; the overall experience of living together was not one I wished to repeat in a hurry. My heart sank at the thought of giving up the privacy of this beautiful house and garden (although it did belong in-tandem to my relatives) and there was nothing I could do but make the best of the situation. I greeted my mother-in-law cheerfully and began helping her to settle in. If I am entirely truthful however, my heart was not in it.

The weeks flew by and soon it was time for my sister-in-law and her family to join us in the big house. Once this happened, there would be nine people sharing the accommodations and whilst normally we all got on well, there were considerations which began to put pressure on the normal harmony which prevailed. My sister-in-law and her husband had a son with a disability and they were still learning to deal with the challenges which a child like this presented on a daily basis. This was the very reason why they had decided to co-habitat with my mother-in-law so she could help them. He was often disturbed by loud noises and would scream uncontrollably when he heard the vacuum cleaner. Change was the thing which disturbed him the most and here was change staring him in the face, not only in the form of a new house but new living companions as well.

My two daughters had a cat called Max whom they adored and who was living with us at the house. Unfortunately my nephew did not like cats and spent the whole time chasing it and trying to catch it, much to my daughters' and the cat's dismay. My mother-in-law, whilst she had been a blessing in the past for my sister and brother-in-law in that she helped them enormously with their son's care, had never lived with him for long periods and found some of his unpredictable behavior beginning to grate on her nerves, especially under these crowded circumstances.

My husband and I had been urged to take the master bedroom while waiting for the arrival of my sister and brother-in-law. When that eventually did happen, they insisted that we remain where we were as they added,

"Your own new house will be finished soon and the changes could happen then."

Unfortunately our building project was experiencing a few quirks of its own as it coincided with a slight recession in the economy and many construction companies were experiencing financial difficulties. Our construction company was no exception. The tradesmen who had been waiting to be paid for some weeks were losing patience and in order to force their employer's hand, began to sabotage our new house. They put rubble in the drains, installed the wiring incorrectly and only raked half the brickwork; something which was expensive and difficult to remedy.

In the meantime, our little shop had its grand opening. Champagne was served, the press arrived and each invited friend and influential guest, sang its praises. Our photograph appeared in the local newspaper and life seemed brimming with promise. Weeks went by and we were basking in the glow of apparent success when our little partnership began to crack at the seams.

After my day off I would return to find that my sister-in-law had moved a few things around to a style more suited to her taste. After this happened a few times, in a cowardly fashion, instead of broaching the subject with her I would simply return the items to where they were in the first place. This went on for some time without discussion but it soon became apparent that when two strong women got together, something had to give.

When we first decided to go into business, I had agreed to a partnership on the basis that my ideas would also be the driving force behind the choice of stock and design. My sister-in-law had initially agreed to this, but as her own creative juices began to bubble forth, she naturally wanted to have an equal say in the input and design and whilst our choices appeared similar in the first instance, there were differences in approach emerging which began to bother me.

Our two husbands could not see what the problem was. The business was, in their opinion, a 'little interest' which their wives had undertaken together and as such, encouraged us to go with the flow. I, on the other hand saw it as my dream of creating something which I could not only deeply relate to but an expression of who I was and was beginning to understand that my sister-in-law and I were on very different pages in that regard.

I began to contemplate just how I could find a peaceful way out of this predicament. It soon presented itself in the guise of my friend whose husband was a master jeweller, trading in one of the more prestigious areas in Eastern Sydney. She told me about a shop for rent a few doors up from theirs. The rent was cheap and the location ideal for the kind of goods we sold. The current site of our little shop on the other hand, whilst conveniently located, had been largely ignored by much of the public who frequented the area. The stock which was beautiful and classic, appealed to a very small section of the population in that it was high-profile and out of character with the normal retail shopping providers in the area.

I jumped at the opportunity to relocate. Not only was it a way to happily dissolve the design differences which we were experiencing, but a way to freely control how the business was run; at least from the second shop. The deal was done, the stock ordered and a second opening celebration held and whilst the extended family came, they were very subdued. Unfazed by this development, I threw myself into the running of my new business. People responded enthusiastically, not only to my personal approach but also to the product and during my first Christmas of trading at the new location, customers were twelve deep at the counter.

My sister-in-law continued to run the first shop and as she was now free to do it her way, things seemed ideal on the surface. Her son however had been experiencing some emotional highs and lows which were disturbing his teacher at school and it soon became clear that his mother running the shop single-handed was not in his best interests. I asked my daughter Penny to help out and she began to relieve at the first shop a few days a week so my sister-in-law could be with her son more often. Regretfully however, she decided that she would have to leave the business altogether and offered to do the book-work instead. This was a blow but her son was a special little boy and I did not wish to be doing anything which would make his life more difficult than it already was. My daughter stepped into the role full time and we ran the two businesses in tandem.

As the weeks wore on, life on the home front began to deteriorate. My once helpful mother-in-law seemed to have jumped camps and whilst my husband was doing everything he could to hurry the building process of our new home, relationships were becoming strained all round. The months slipped by and as the stress of our home situation grew worse, I noticed that my neck was now swollen on both sides.

Of course I was so busy with the two shops that I barely had time to cope with my daily chores, let alone examine my neck. Not only had the original lumps increased, but I also discovered lumps under my arms as well. The disease had gone into forward gear.

Sandra Munro

Chapter Four

Decisions

Only peace can remove you from chaos.
The Keys of Joshua — Glenda Green

The faces of the panel of ten specialists who sat around the table were serious. It was usual at the hospital for these experts to examine the evidence and make pronouncements and I was about to receive mine.

"The disease has progressed dramatically", they spoke in hushed tones. "It is our opinion that you should proceed with intense Chemotherapy and Radiation at the earliest possible moment, as we feel you have less than three months left to live".

I was not even sure what I was feeling at that moment. My mind was in turmoil. Three months! How is that possible? It was only a few months ago that they were telling me that I had years. What had changed? Deep down however, I knew. Things at home were a mess, the building of our home was in chaos, and now my health ... well, it didn't bear thinking about. The thoughts went round and round in my head. I had to say something. They were all waiting, then it struck me. I didn't want to have that treatment, it felt wrong; somehow I would find another way.

I opened my mouth to speak and they all sat waiting patiently and sympathetically for my response.

"I don't want to have that treatment". I spoke with all the conviction I could muster.

"I am going to try some alternate treatments and see how I go. I might agree to have it later, but not now", I couldn't believe what I heard myself saying but I stuck to my guns. "That is my decision".

The specialists looked at one another,

"Well", the spokesperson said "I wouldn't wait too long. This is very serious you understand".

I nodded my head and clutching tight to my husband's hand, left the room. I had no idea how I was going to do this, or even if it would work. I knew nothing about Cancer but I could feel the stubbornness rise in my belly. I was going to give it my best shot!

On the way to work the next morning, I left early and took a different route, as I wanted to take down the Christmas Tree which was still in the shop window in order to give the shop a fresh new look. This task was just the distraction I needed to keep my mind off the doctors' diagnosis. As I put my foot down slowly on the accelerator to move forward in the traffic, out of the corner of my eye I saw a car run the red light on the opposite side of the road and, missing the first two cars, plough into the front of mine with terrifying intensity. Shaken but seemingly not hurt, I got out of the car, which was now immobilized and approached the driver who had stopped and was shaking in his seat.

"What were you doing?" I asked him, "driving through a red light like that?"

"I'm so sorry" he said, "I misread the light signal which showed a left-turn arrow and went straight ahead. Are you alright?" he asked.

"I'm fine", I responded, realizing that apart from some shaking, I really was fine. "I think we should go to the Police Station, it is just around the corner from here," I said.

The other driver agreed and took off. As my car was in no fit state to drive at that moment, I had to walk around the corner to the police station. I moved more slowly than usual as I was still shaking from the impact and it took me a few moments to arrive. When I entered the station, I saw the other driver completing his statement of events.

The officer at the counter greeted me curtly when I explained that I was the second driver in the incident. She asked me to take a breath test, as it seemed it had already been explained to the police that I was the culprit who ran the red light. Indignantly I tried to explain my position and became very upset in the process.

"Now I understand", I blurted out, "When you are in the wrong you just lie and the police believe you and the innocent party is left holding the bag".

The policewoman stared at me in a startled manner.

"Well if you are going to give me a breath test, you had better give him one as well. We need to keep it fair." I said. When this was done, it was discovered that the other driver had a high alcohol reading due to a party he had attended the previous evening. No apologies were offered, but I felt justified nevertheless. Wasn't there enough happening in my life at the moment without a driver lying about his part in a road accident? I called my husband to have the car towed away and wondered at life's complications.

In the meantime I had to refine my search for some alternate ways to heal and began to scour the bookshops for anything in print which would give me a clue. As

chance would have it my husband was about to partici-
pate in a sailing regatta in a lovely coastal town north of
where we lived. Although I didn't sail, I went along and
while he was out competing on the water, I was exploring
the local bookshops for anything likely to help my situation. I was about to give up my search as fruitless, when
my eye suddenly caught a rainbow on the cover of a book
called You Can Heal Your Life by an American woman
called Louise Hay. It seems she had cured herself of Cancer through the use of the techniques set out in the book. I
placed it resolutely on the counter. Now I was getting
somewhere.

The book was written in an easy style, although the
content was far from familiar. Louise it seems was promoting a sense of gratitude for everything in your life and
while that made sense; thanking your refrigerator, your
bed and your car was a little out of my league; nevertheless I kept on reading because this woman had actually
cured herself without medical intervention and there was
nothing more motivating than the example of someone

who has succeeded in the very thing you are trying to accomplish.

The second book I discovered was written by an Australian medical doctor, Ainsley Meers, who in his efforts to help his Cancer patients had employed the use of meditation with pleasing results. Unfortunately Dr. Meers had recently died which ruled out having a personal conversation and left me with only his scant research to cling to.

As chance would have it my husband's secretary had recently had surgery for a malignant condition in her Thyroid and he asked her if she would call me and discuss her experience. Kate was a fiery redhead and a very practical person, however when challenged with such a serious illness, had decided in part to embrace an alternate course of therapy to support her medical treatment. Kate told me that she had taken a series of Colonic Irrigations; a procedure which cleanses the bowel and promotes a more efficient uptake of nutrients, apparently a valuable benefit when you were fighting a serious disease. I listened quietly and when she hung up, decided that I would give this a try.

I found the practitioner's office and sat waiting in the little room set aside for this purpose. The walls were lined with illustrations of human internal organs and charts depicting an enlarged diagram of a human iris. It all felt strange and unfamiliar and I almost got up and went home. While I was trying to make up my mind, a cheery woman, dressed in a nurse's uniform called my name and beckoned me into a cubicle where the procedure was to take place.

The woman sensed my anxiety and continued to chat about everyday things, telling me that she worked at the local hospital. She was soon joined by a small man with a goatee (something which made him seem slightly questionable in my mind) and who began to look into my eyes for an extended period. I was quite put out by this invasion of my privacy and asked him what he was doing.

"I am looking into your eyes to determine what I can discover there," he answered. "It is a practice known as Iridology and it can tell me a great deal about what your body is doing at this current point in time".

He went on to explain that there seemed to be a problem with my spleen and that the condition of this organ was indicating a serious illness. I told him about the diagnosis and he nodded his head adding, "Ah yes, the spleen is one of the organs most likely to indicate such a condition". At this time I had no idea that my spleen was involved in my illness and it wasn't until later, that this was confirmed for me by the doctor. In some instances of this disease, the spleen is actually removed in the hope that it will somehow improve the condition.

The practitioner in the meantime, pressed on with the Colonic Irrigation which, whilst not painful was decidedly uncomfortable and I decided that this was the last time I would undergo such a procedure. The nurse in an effort to calm my angst, continued to chat and the topic of

Meditation came up. She told me that there was a Professor of Surgery at the local teaching hospital who could put a whole room of people into meditation within a few moments.

Driving home in the car I began to wonder about Iridology and how strange it was that just by looking into people's eyes, problems in the body could be detected. I also thought about the Professor and meditation and decided to give him a call the following day. I rang first thing in the morning and discovered that he ran a special meditation class for Cancer patients, which was held at the local teaching hospital. Unfortunately it was earlier than the time I closed the shop and I enquired if they were held at any other time. The Professor confirmed that they were also held at another Centre and after writing down the details, I decided to go.

Louise Hay had recommended making a list of those people in your life you felt needed forgiving for some perceived slight, or even in certain cases, someone who had done something so serious that in Louise's opinion;

must be forgiven without delay. I knew many such people; my father being one case in particular and one with whom I had locked horns on more than one occasion. My husband had also presented some problems over time, causing me to doubt his commitment on occasion. Yet lately, since my diagnosis, he had been almost the perfect husband, attending my every need and I was feeling especially contented while basking in this care.

An even more gloomy memory was my relative who, when I was a child, had touched me inappropriately over a number of years. Even though I hadn't spoken of this to anyone, or even thought about him or his actions for years, I obviously needed to consider forgiving him as well. Of course Louise was not recommending you needed to do this in person; just writing down the names and bringing the person and incident to mind and having the intention to do so, did the trick.

I began at once and the list seemed to get longer and longer as I thought about the hurtful way teachers, friends and colleagues had treated me over the years. Yet Louise had also suggested that forgiving yourself was equally important, so, retracing my steps, I began again; this time bringing to mind those I had slighted and treated badly and this was a much more sobering activity, as I recalled time after time when I had been thoughtless or selfish, hurting those I cared about; even though on most occasions it was unintentional.

This was ongoing work and as each day dawned, some new memory would present itself for my attention. In addition, Louise suggested beginning a programme which addressed how you felt about yourself. Did you approve of yourself; liking the way you looked or moved or behaved? I had no doubts on that score. I was always unhappy with how I looked, but despite changing my heritage, could not see what I could do about that.

Louise however had other ideas. She advocated an affirmation as often as possible, proclaiming that you ap-proved of yourself and although I could not see what possible use this could be, I began and whenever I thought of it, would repeat it to myself over and over again.

Chapter Five

Shifting

When you do the inner work,

You are eternally forgiven.

The Awakening — Hanneke Jennings

As I awoke one morning, I climbed out of bed and padded to the window. A slight drizzle was smearing the windowpane and picking up my swimsuit, I went into the bathroom to wash my face; and then gazed into the mirror as I mouthed my affirmations. I ran down the stairs and out through the kitchen into the garden, when my mother-in-law, who was by the sink washing dishes; called after me,

"You are not going for a swim today are you? It is such a horrible day."

I pretended I had not heard and tried not to let the words touch me as I slipped into the deep end of the pool. Rolling onto my back and letting the gentle rain moisten my face, I stroked leisurely backwards towards the other end.

"Why did some people feel the need to spoil such a simple pleasure", I wondered? It was after all, only rain. Concentrating on my backstroke for several more laps, I eventually pulled myself out and sat on the steps, enjoying the feeling of energy flowing through my body. Perhaps my mother-in-law's negativity was caused by looking forward to spending some private time here at her new home. I felt contrite and picked up my towel to retrace my steps. I would make amends and offer to help her with the washing up.

As I stepped back into the kitchen, my mother-in-law continued as if the conversation had not been interrupted.

"As I was saying" she said with some emphasis, "Why would anyone even want to go into the pool on such a day?" I swallowed in an effort to control my response.

"Actually it was really lovely in the water, in spite of the rain", I said evenly.

Not convinced, my mother-in-law turned her back and dipping her hands into the suds, went on with the washing up.

Maintaining equilibrium in the face of such a lack of enthusiasm was proving to be something of a task, but hadn't Louise Hay said that we had to replace those disapproving thoughts which plagued us with more positive and supportive ones. With this in mind, I climbed the stairs repeating softly to myself, I approve of myself; everything in my life is perfect.

The first evening of the meditation course was looming and I realized that it coincided with my daughter Penny's twenty-first birthday.

"We can't possibly go that evening" I told my husband.

"Penny would hate it."

He tightened his jaw,

"We are going." he said. "She will understand."

Penny of course was aware of my illness and was being very supportive, relieving me at the shop as much as she could when my energy levels dropped, but it was fast becoming clear that the two shops could not continue to operate for much longer and I had begun to make plans to close the original business. This was a worrying prospect as the stock had to be relocated and as the lease was still operating, there would be payments to attend to without income to support them.

The evening of the Meditation class finally arrived and we all drove the few miles to the Centre which was located in a small side street in a suburb I had not visited since I was a child. As we drove in past the high walls, a small sign announced that we were entering the Meditation Centre. After parking the car in the rear garden, we were greeted by two women with smiling faces who welcomed us warmly.

"Please remove your shoes and place them in the pigeon holes provided," the two women beamed at us.

"Why do we need to take off our shoes?" I wondered as I sought out a pigeon hole which provided just the right space for them.

After my husband and two daughters had removed their shoes, we all padded in bare feet towards the area where the women had indicated that the Meditation Class would take place. Moving down the corridor, I looked at large photographs of people dressed in what appeared to be Indian garb. There was one photograph in particular which portrayed the face of a young boy, although he looked so beautiful he could be a woman.

"If angels were human", this person would definitely be one" I thought and as I moved off down the corridor, the beautiful eyes seemed to smile at me.

The Professor was already in the room setting up the technical equipment and on the floor was a musical instrument which looked like a piano accordion. There were also more of the smiling women to greet us and show us to our places. The room was half-filled with people, who were also there with their families and I wondered which of them had Cancer.

The professor introduced himself and the evening began with a series of slides which depicted the disease in its many forms. This was the first time that I had been confronted with such hard evidence and my heart lurched as I watched. It was one thing to imagine that I could defeat this inner enemy with alternate means and quite another to see its progress depicted so graphically.

The Professor invited a man who was sitting right in front of me to take the podium. He was tall, much the same age as my husband and he spoke about his wife, the progress of her Cancer and the benefits of Meditation. I listened intently so as to absorb every word. Then he said something which rocked me to my core.

"Unfortunately my wife did not make it." I heard him say.

"Did I hear correctly?" "Surely that was his young attractive wife sitting right there next to him?"

No, I had heard correctly, the man was actually telling all those who had come here filled with hope, that despite the Meditation, his wife had died.

I felt the anger rise in my belly.

"What was the point of all this?" Why bother to bring people here at all?"

I wanted to get up and leave right then. I had really thought that there was a way, but here was someone saying that even this way was doubtful. Before I could move however, the lights dimmed and the Professor drew our attention to a sign at the front of the room. On it were written the words Om Namah Shivaya. As the anger was still bubbling within me, I could not even read them properly. I tried to speak them to myself silently, but for some reason they just would not compute and no matter how hard I tried, they would fly out of my mind like quicksilver and I had to glue my eyes to the letters to even pronounce them.

The professor explained that the words were in Sanskrit, a very ancient Indian language and they meant: I honor the Self within. Well, I thought, at least that was a little bit like approving of yourself and wasn't this important? I began to try to focus, although the words still would not stay in my mind and I had to repeat them over and over again just to keep them in my awareness.

The Professor sat on the floor and began to play the musical instrument which resembled a piano-accordion and as he did so, he began to sing these same words in a strange and haunting melody. He encouraged those in the hall to repeat each phrase after him and told us that this practice was called chanting and that these sounds were very beneficial for the body.

I found that the words (which kept sliding out of my mind) and the strange sound of the chant only heightened my sense of rising alarm as I wondered what I was doing here. As the sound of the chant faded, the Professor gently led us into Meditation, encouraging us to continue to repeat the words Om Namah Shivaya to ourselves on the in-breath and again on the out-breath. I closed my eyes and could hear the sounds of the people in the room as if they were magnified. Every breath seemed larger than life and there were various coughing, snuffling and bodily movements as people settled into the process. On the other hand, I didn't seem to be able to do this Meditation thing at all. It seemed no time at all however, before the professor was gently asking us to bring our awareness back to the room and telling us to open our eyes.

Afterwards, he asked people to share their experience and many spoke of feeling as though they had no body; or had glimpsed a vast night sky, complete with stars; or even the perfect stillness of nothingness. I completely related to this last response. I had felt nothing at all. Afterwards they served tea and although I sought out the man who had spoken about his dead wife, he was nowhere to be found. I wanted to speak to him as my anger still buzzed in my belly like a hive of bees.

This evening had been an introduction and the real Learn to Meditate Course began the following week. I was not sure if I wanted to go. The following morning, the image of the man who spoke about his wife dying of Cancer was the first thought in my head when I awoke. I needed to talk to him. Perhaps all was not as it seemed and there might be something positive to be gained after all. I rang the Meditation Centre to see if I could find out how to contact the man. He answered the telephone.

As I spoke with him, to my embarrassment I found myself in tears. What was the matter with me? He told me that he would be in for the rest of the day as he was doing some work, seva he called it (which I later learned meant selfless service) at the Centre. I agreed to drive over and meet with him.

When I arrived, James which I learned was his name, was waiting for me at the front desk. He was answering the phones. He took a break and we retired to the tearoom to make a cup of tea. He promised to lend me some books which might make sense of things and told me a little of the story of his wife's illness. He seemed to be at peace with the outcome but as we spoke, I could feel the fear rising in my throat. All this talk of death made me jumpy. James promised to drop the books off to me at the shop the next day and as I walked slowly back to my car, I felt relieved to be driving back home where I could feel 'normal' again.

Its all about Love

Chapter Six

Choices

If you want good health, you

must endeavor to live your

life in harmony with the divine

Law of Love.

White Eagle on the Great Spirit

The following day at the shop I was sorting out some stock when a young woman entered and approached me. She handed me a leaflet which was advertising a Meditation class run by a person called Petrea King and wondered if I would be interested in attending. I marveled at the coincidence but told the woman I had only signed up the previous evening for just such a course. The woman asked me the name of the organization and on learning what it was said,

"Do you know what *that* is all about?" I asked her what she meant.

"Well, it is a very different kind of meditation" the woman went on. "I just thought you should know" and with that she left the shop.

Afterward I pondered her remarks. What did she mean by a different kind of meditation? Not long afterwards, James entered the shop carrying a pile of books and despite my previous reaction, I was pleased to see him, if only to get an answer to my question. He listened carefully and nodded his head.

"Oh she is talking about the lineage" he responded.

"They have a meditation Master who heads up the organization, some refer to her as a Guru. There is a large photograph of her in the foyer, didn't you notice it when you were there?" he asked.

I had noticed a large photograph of what I thought was a beautiful young boy. This, it seemed was the Guru, taken just after she had cut her hair, a common practice with Swamis. I remembered thinking what a gentle and loving face she had and wished I had taken more notice. James went on to tell me that the Swami, known affectionately as Gurumayi or Guru Mother, lived between her two Ashrams in India and Upstate New York.

After putting the books down on the counter, he turned to leave and said he would watch out for me when I next came to the Centre and to be sure to call him if I had any further questions. After he had left I found it difficult to keep my mind on my work. Thoughts of Ashrams and Gurus were floating about in my head and I wondered what I had gotten myself into.

The following week soon arrived and my family, minus my eldest daughter who decided she wanted nothing more to do with meditation; piled into the car for the short drive to the Centre. This time the class was held in a smaller room at the back of the building and when we entered, there was a circle of about twelve people sitting on the floor waiting for the session to begin. The professor arrived and the chanting began. I still couldn't believe how difficult it was to remember the phrase *Om Namah Shivaya.* Normally my mind was razor sharp and my memory excellent, but on this occasion something odd seemed to be happening.

After a short period of chanting, the professor led the group into meditation and when the bell rang to bring us out of our reverie, I was surprised to note that almost fifteen minutes had passed. It seemed shorter and although I had still experienced nothing significant, the time had certainly flown. Afterwards as we gathered again in the tea room for cake and conversation, people crowded around the professor with questions about how to perfect their meditation technique and others just began to chat quietly.

I was standing with my husband and youngest daughter, who was just sixteen and wide-eyed at the unfamiliar surroundings, when two women approached. One of them was wearing a headscarf which signified that she had lost her hair due to Chemotherapy and the other, who was accompanied by a friend, had a slight limp. I discovered that they were about my age and were both experiencing different kinds of Cancer. As we wished each other goodnight, we agreed to talk more the following week.

Several weeks went by and the meditation classes progressed fairly uneventfully. The routine was always the same, sitting in a circle, sharing something of note which had happened during the week, a short chant and then into the meditation, which gradually increased to a full half hour. Although the meditation sessions were not developing dramatically, I wished I could say the same for my disease, which seemed to have jumped into forward gear. My lymph nodes continued to enlarge until I looked as though I was several months pregnant with a double case of the Mumps and the X-rays were indicating that the Cancer had metastasized and was beginning to infiltrate my vital organs. Why wasn't anything working?

Each night when I would fall into bed, I would experience a dull ache which intensified over time, causing my husband to have to rub my back continually to allow me to get even short periods of sleep. I had streamlined my diet, mainly eating vegetables, fruit and grains and was drinking fresh juices combined with large spoonfuls of a powder blend called *Green Magma.* This looked and tasted like green talcum powder but was said to do wonders for the body.

My illness had finally kept me from the shop and as my daughter Penny took care of the business on her own, I stayed at home each day trying to visualize myself as a lithe young woman with long flowing hair loping along the beach in the sunshine. Each day when I sat for meditation, I would bring this image into my mind, refining it endlessly and making my body slimmer and healthier (a far cry from the way I looked at the time). I saw my face as more beautiful (without the lumps) and would picture my hair as silky and blonde swinging in the breeze and my body tanned and slender; at the peak of fitness. I could almost feel the sand between my toes and hear the gentle sound of the waves as they rolled up the beach.

I had learned this technique from a book called *Creative Visualization* by Shakti Gawain and became so attached to this alter ego, that I almost came to believe that this was who I really was. I had also read that a similar technique was being used with children diagnosed with Leukemia, where they pretended that their cancer cells were aliens which they 'shot down and eliminated' in the manner of a computer game.

Soon the pain was too severe for me to drive and to make matters worse, one of my friends at the Meditation class had gone into hospital, with her doctors suggesting that she had only a week or two left to live. I went to see her but despite the fact that she understood the situation; I couldn't seem to find the right words. As a result we avoided the subject of her illness altogether and spoke of her children and the funny things they were doing and the mischief they got up to when they came to visit their mother in the hospital and surprisingly, we were able to laugh together.

With death staring us both in the face, it was a kind of release. My friend died quietly and I rang her husband and offered my sympathies but it felt hollow. Would I be next? I didn't know; in fact I didn't know much at all anymore. Nothing seemed to be able to penetrate the wall I was building around myself.

The house was finally finished but by the time the removal date rolled around and after nearly eight months of close co-habitation, the atmosphere between our two families was very strained. As time was running out for me, my husband was determined that I would enjoy my new home while I could, however not long after we moved in, we noticed that there was a problem with one of the walls in the living room and it was necessary for the tradesmen to return to repair it. In order to do this, they needed to bring cement into the house in a wheel-barrow over the new cream carpet.

This latest problem was taking its toll on my emotions. Of course it was not just the building but the disease which was not responding to my best efforts despite meditation, diet, visualization and positive affirmations. It just seemed to be galloping full steam ahead.

Its all about Love

Chapter Seven

Shaving

When your habitual thinking

is harmonious and constructive,

you experience perfect health ...

The Power of Your Subconscious Mind — Joseph Murphy

My husband, always resourceful, had a great idea.

"I will just put down some plastic sheets and tape them to the carpet and once the workers have left, we will pull it all up again and it will be as good as new".

I agreed and my husband in his thorough way, began to tape down the sheets. He brought some tape from work but it was bright orange and before long the house was littered with strips of orange tape.

The workers came, the job was done and together we proceeded to pull up the plastic. Much to my horror, the orange tape had left corresponding stripes all over the beautiful new cream carpet.

"I am sure it will come off" my husband said.

Unfortunately it did not and the insurance company didn't seem to want to know about it. We had spent all our money and couldn't afford to replace the carpet and it seemed, on the surface, to be another calamity.

Coincidentally a friend of ours knew someone who worked at the company which manufactured the carpet and they had suggested taking a stained piece and putting it under a microscope to see how deeply the colour had penetrated the fibers. We arranged this and fortunately, the penetration was only minimal. Our friend then came up with another great idea.

"Why don't you shave it off", he suggested. We had nothing to lose; by this stage of my illness I was feeling quite weak and had to sit down from time to time to conserve my energy and as I was no longer at work, it would give me something to focus on. My husband went out and bought several packets of razors and I began.

Even though the stains were disappearing in response to the shaving, I had to grit my teeth with determination each morning as I thought of kneeling on the soft carpet and shaving yet another patch. The only consolation was that from time to time I would lie on the soft, velvety carpet, close my eyes and do my visualization. This time however, I saw myself shaving in fast forward and the stains disappearing as if by magic.

My friend Kathy came to my rescue and lent me a tape by an American motivator called *Zig Ziglar* who, in his twanging Southern drawl recommended

"Never giving up before you reach the goal" and to *"Keep on keeping on"*.

As I listened to the burley Texan it kept up my spirits and just when I felt ready to give up, I would be inspired to shave yet another patch.

The series of meditation classes with the Professor was almost finished and my husband's company had instructed him to go to Edinburgh on business for a week. He wondered if I felt up to going with him. I loved the soft green countryside in the north of England, although I had never been to Scotland before and even began to think that perhaps I had better join him in case this was the last time I would see this green and pleasant land. A few months earlier this thought would not have even crossed my mind but the disease was stubbornly refusing to co-operate and I had even begun contemplating taking some chemotherapy; if I hadn't left it too late.

One day as I lay on the carpet taking a rest, I started to feel the anger rising up into my throat. Why wasn't anything working? What did I have to do to make it happen? Why did I have to shave the carpet every day and pretend that I was lithe and lovely and running on the beach? In my mind I shouted to whoever was listening in the stillness,

"What's it all about?" To my surprise, and as if in response to my question, a clear voice replied,

"It's all about love". Startled I looked around but knew that there was no one there. The voice had been in my head. Was I going mad as well? Perhaps this was a symptom of my deteriorating health? Somehow though, I didn't think so.

Chapter Eight

The Green and Pleasant Land

Go into the country, lean with your back

against a tree trunk and listen to the song

of the wind and the rustle of the leaves.

It has a message for you . . .

White Eagle on the Great Spirit

The flight from Australia to London seemed longer than usual and I was tired when we arrived. My husband had decided to drive north instead of taking the flight to Edinburgh so that we could enjoy the scenery and had arranged a hire car at the airport. As we turned on to the freeway, a slight rain began to fall and the hum of the motor lulled me into a daydream. I smiled to myself and wondered how long it would take to drive to Edinburgh. It was a relief to let go and think of nothing and as the rows of houses gave way to green fields, I soon fell into a dreamless sleep.

When I awoke we were driving through the Border Counties and we stopped at a small lodge so we could take some refreshment. The landscape was sparser than that around London, and the architecture of the small building was Spartan. This I guessed, signaled that we were already in Scotland and as my husband helped me out of the car and I walked the few steps to the door of the Lodge, I could smell the aroma of lunch.

Vegetarianism seemed almost unheard of in this part of Scotland. The menu consisted of baked meats, grilled meats and stewed meats with lashings of vegetables on the side. I went for the vegetables, even though they were more than thoroughly cooked; followed by a tinned juice. Later as we walked through the hall of the Lodge, marveling at its pristine cleanliness and threadbare carpet, I began to understand why the Scots were so frugal.

Throughout history, times had been hard for these brave people and living here, in the Border Counties could not have been easy. The Lodge must have been at least two hundred years old and I wondered what kind of history the successive owners had endured in their fight to preserve the sanctity of their land. We completed our meal and were soon on the last leg of our journey. As the rows of sparse houses gave way to the grey stone villas on the outskirts of Edinburgh, I began to look forward to a hot shower and a soft, warm bed.

The hotel where my husband was booked to have his business meeting was unimposing, although the polished wood of the front desk and the shining old fashioned brass bell brought the promise of good old fashioned service. We were soon settled into our room which, although sustaining the frugality of my first impressions of Scotland, did not disappoint and later that evening as I climbed into the crisp sheets and began my affirmations silently in my head, despite the nagging ache in my body; I was soon deeply asleep.

My husband's business complete, he had decided to surprise me and take a longer route south via the beautiful Lakes District in Cumbria and as our little car climbed through the bare mountains adjoining this jewel in England's crown, and as we stopped every now and again for a lost black-faced sheep who had wandered onto the road, I began to look forward to something for the first time in months.

I had heard about The Lakes District since I was a child as it had once been the home of the famed Beatrix Potter, authoress of the series of children's classics called *Peter Rabbit and Friends* and beloved by my own children, who had insisted on collecting the whole series and despite being grown now, still kept them among their favourites.

On the drive down through the mountains towards the string of lakes at their base, the beauty of the landscape was breathtaking. Quaint houses with thatched roofs were set amidst spectacular gardens and as it was early Spring, the crisp air seemed to make everything sparkle. I sighed; if this was indeed my last trip abroad, I could not have wished for anything better.

As the houses began to cluster together I realized that we must be entering the picturesque town of Windemere, with its charming slate-roofed hotels and cobbled streets. We soon found one which appealed to our idea of the perfect place to stay and after a delicious dinner in the small dining room, where we were eyed curiously by the other guests; we were soon settled in a small room tucked under the eaves. It was all the proprietor could offer as the town was filling up with tourists who came for the astonishing display of nature at that time of year. As we huddled down beneath our quilt, I sighed with contentment, hardly noticing the familiar deep ache in my body.

In the morning my husband asked me if I was up to taking a walk down to the Lake. We took it slowly, pausing every now and then for me to catch my breath. The descent was gentle and wound through a wood filled with trees whose lime green buds were pregnant with the promise of the season. The ground was carpeted with Bluebells and Cowslips, which appeared almost iridescent in the gentle beams of sunlight filtering down through the branches. The path was strewn with the fallen leaves of Autumn which settled into a brown softness underfoot and as we paused for a break, out of the corner of my eye I spied the burnished amber coat of that diminishing species; the Red Squirrel.

In that moment, time stood still as I breathed in the beauty of this place. It only lasted a second, like a frozen frame in a movie and yet it was timeless and as I began to move my feet again, the natural sounds and movement of the woods resumed and I wondered if I had somehow imagined the frozen beauty I had just witnessed.

Its all about Love

Chapter Nine

A Stitch In Time Saves Nine

Once a chick has emerged from its

shell or a butterfly from its chrysalis,

there is no going back...

Opening Doors Within – Eileen Caddy

Back in Australia again, I resumed my sessions at the Meditation class. I now had to loosen my clothing to sit, as my stomach was very distended due to my illness and as I struggled to find a comfortable position in which to meditate, I tried to surrender to the process, closing my eyes and hoping to find that still, quiet place within. My mind however was having none of it and stubbornly began to recall scenes from our recent overseas trip.

One scene in particular kept flashing forth in my mind and as I tried in vain to block it out, it grew in intensity; almost as if I was actually there in those woods carpeted with Bluebells and gazing in rapt attention at the beautiful red squirrel. It was almost as though I could reach out and touch the gleaming red coat, breathe in the beauty of the lime green leaf tips and hear the soft squish of the leaves underfoot.

The intensity of the experience was extraordinary and I wondered if I could recall other memories in the same vivid way. No sooner had I had this thought than I was airborne, seemingly out of my body and flying over the river near my former home. I looked down and saw the whole scene as though I was a bird; distinguishing the outdoor furniture by the pool and the Camellias in full bloom in the garden. Was this a memory, I wondered? Then I realized that this was not *my* outdoor furniture; it actually belonged to the new owner of the property. This was happening *now*. What was this all about?

Softly the bell chimed to bring us out of meditation and as I opened my eyes I wondered at what had just happened. The others got up to leave and I remained behind, leaning against the wall. The professor came over to see if everything was alright. I explained what had happened. He smiled and told me that this was a good thing and sometimes occurred in meditation. He explained that there was going to be a fuller session of meditation held at the centre over the weekend.

"Why don't you think about attending?" he queried.

On the way home I was still thinking about my unusual meditation experience and thought,

"What harm can it do, nothing else seems to be working!".

The day of the meditation dawned bright and clear. A friend picked me up as I was no longer able to drive the car and drove my youngest daughter, Melanie and me to the Centre. At sixteen, Melanie had embraced meditation and everything to do with it wholeheartedly and was very excited about going. On the other hand, I seemed to have slipped into a rather unusual state of mind. As I loosened my clothing and took my seat in the hall, I began to take a mental note the number of people there. There was a small charge for the programme, and I began to calculate how much money the centre would be taking on the day. Some part of me was refusing to believe that this could do any good. What was I doing here?

The program began and the first meditation unfolded uneventfully and as I struggled to keep my eyes closed, disturbed not only by the noises in the room but by my physical discomfort, I was glad when the bell rang to bring us out of our reverie. Moving out into the sunshine, I sipped my tea and chatted to my friends from the Cancer group.

Soon it was time to return to the hall which was dimmed and quiet and as I loosened my clothing and settled into the most comfortable position I could find, I was tempted to leave but before I could get up, the harmonium began to play the strains of **Om Namah Shivaya** and the words of the chant began to soothe me and, closing my eyes, I finally surrendered to the process.

After what seemed like a few minutes, the room seemed to become several shades darker and a strange vibration began to move up through my body which soon began to rock to and fro, gently at first and then more and more violently. This new development was accompanied by large hot tears which rolled incessantly down my cheeks forming sodden puddles on my collar. The crying was silent at first then huge wracking sobs jolted my body as I was shaking and rocking and sobbing all at once.

My daughter Melanie who was sitting beside me became embarrassed,

"Mum" she whispered into the darkness, "Shhh! People can hear you."

I did not know what was happening but I knew that I had absolutely no control over it. At the side of the hall, two hall monitors were watching me quietly. They were used to unusual things happening in Meditation Intensives, for that is indeed what this was. They were going to keep an eye on me.

Suddenly I felt a sharp pain at the base of my abdomen, as though someone had plunged a knife deep in my belly and was dragging it upwards towards my chest. The shock of the pain, coupled with the dragging sensation, caused me to hyperventilate in an effort to control my panic. I cried out silently in my mind to make it stop. I even had to admit the possibility that I might be dying right here in the hall, after all the disease was certainly getting worse and my pain levels were intolerable on occasion. I was abysmally ignorant about the progress of the disease; what you did not know couldn't hurt you, I had figured. This was certainly an 'ostrich with its head in the sand' kind of attitude but it had worked for me so far; or so I thought.

Then I had another thought. Didn't the Professor say that you would never be given anything you couldn't handle in meditation? Perhaps this was a meditation experience? No sooner had I contemplated this idea than perience? No sooner had I contemplated this idea than the pain began to subside, only to be replaced by a sensation of falling backwards head first down a deep dark hole. Initially it happened in slow motion and the sensation was quite pleasurable but then my fall began to accelerate and the panic set in again as I was plummeting head first, further and further into the darkness. Trying to get my mind around what was happening I called silently, yet urgently into the void for it to *"Stop!"*

No sooner had this thought been expressed than my fall was immediately halted and I hung suspended in the velvety blackness, swinging gently to and fro as if cocooned in a soft hammock. The feeling was quite incredible; a sensation of such tenderness and safety that all fear dissipated. My cells seemed to be opening like flowers to the rain. It was indescribably beautiful; as though love was embracing every cell of my being and making it whole. The experience was exquisite and I wondered if perhaps if I had died after all. If so, I was content to remain where I was forever.

I have no idea how long I remained in that beautiful place. There seemed to be no time; but eventually a soft tinkling sound began to permeate my reverie. It was the bell to bring us out of meditation. I struggled to open my eyes but they seemed glued shut. Finally I opened them and tried to stand up, but my legs felt like jelly and I staggered and fell back. Quickly the hall monitors hurried to assist me, helping me out of the hall into the sunshine where they sat me on a stool and brought me a cup of hot tea to revive me.

Sandra Munro

Chapter Ten

Feathers and Other Miracles

When you experience deep contentment,

you are able to allow the sacred power, whose nature

is supreme bliss, to shine forth.

Courage and Contentment

A Collection of Talks on Spiritual Life – Gurumayi Chidvilasanda

After the meditation experience I sought out the Professor and shared what had happened. He listened most intently and suggested that I share it with a lady who was sitting in the tearoom. I wondered at this suggestion as I had never met the woman before but obliged him and went and introduced myself.

I was still feeling very strange as if I were not quite in my body. The room was crowded and as there was no available seating, I sat on the floor to relate my story. I had just got to the most interesting part when I stopped. Lately when I sat, I had to loosen my clothing as it was uncomfortable for me to sit due to the enlarged nature of my body. Yet here I was, sitting cross-legged on the floor, happily talking to this stranger and yet there was no pain or discomfort at all. What was going on?

The remainder of the day was uneventful by comparison and when I got home I was so tired that I just rolled into bed and before my husband could reach out to massage the pain which was my constant companion, I had fallen into the first deep sleep I had experienced for months.

The following morning, I woke up and jumped out of bed and ran downstairs. It wasn't until I reached the kitchen that I realized what I had done. It had been some time since I could 'jump' or even 'run' anywhere; my energy levels and the pain I was experiencing, had precluded such activity. I turned on the kettle to make some tea and went out into the garden to hose the plants.

As I stepped through the door and gazed at the front lawn, it had a strange, almost iridescent glow. The flowers seemed surreal in their intensity of colour and as I watched a small sparrow which was frolicking in the garden bed, I wondered why I had never noticed the intricacy of colour and pattern in each small feather before; they were almost like miniature works of art. Everything glowed and sparkled and it felt as though I was dreaming. A man walked by the house on his early morning walk and as our eyes met, I experienced such a feeling of pure and innocent love that it took my breath away.

"What was happening to me?" I wondered?

The kettle whistled from the kitchen and as I returned to the house to make the tea and climbed the stairs to take a cup to my husband, (the first in a long time as he was usually the one to bring it to me), I placed it on the bedside table and wondered about my experience.

After much heart-searching I had finally decided to visit the oncologist. I had been trying for months to arrest the progress of the Cancer without success and felt as though I had nothing to lose. My initial consultation was a few days before the Meditation program and the doctor had recommended a course of *soft* chemotherapy; the same chemicals as those given intravenously, but taken in tablet form. Now here I was on the day following my strange Meditation to pick up my prescription and as I waited for my appointment, wondered if my unusual experience would affect the final outcome. The doctor smiled at me gently and wrote out the script, handing it to me and telling me to go to the hospital pharmacy to have it filled. I had already decided that if I was going to take these chemicals, I might as well make a little ceremony out of it and after creating a small altar, replete with a few flowers from the garden, I placed the pills there for a short while. As I affirmed that they were doing me good, I popped them into my mouth with every confidence that this was the truth.

A week or two later I returned to the doctor's office for a check-up and he asked me to climb up on the examination table, where he began to prod the areas where the lumps were most prominent. He prodded and prodded; and then he prodded some more and I was prompted by the strange expression on his face to ask if there was something wrong.

"As a matter of fact there is" he responded. My heart began to thump very loudly. "I can't find anything" the doctor replied.

"What did you say?" I asked, as if not trusting my words.

"I can't find anything. Please get up and I will write you a referral for a scan and a blood test so we can get to the bottom of this." He spoke almost inaudibly and I strained to hear as he wrote out the required script.

The following day as I sat in his office listening to him read out the results of the scan and the blood test, I was astounded. The disease had vanished as if it had never been there. Usually there was scar tissue remaining when patients go into remission but even this remnant was absent on this occasion. It was as though the cancer had melted like ice-cream in the hot sun. Of course, in his conservative way and left without what he considered a logical explanation, the oncologist wanted me to continue with the pills for a while longer and as I walked out of the surgery that day, I was puzzled. What had made this happen? The questions would not leave me and I would lie awake at night wondering how and indeed why, it had occurred.

Of course instead of focusing on the blessing of recovery, understandably perhaps, I could only wonder if the disease which had so mysteriously vanished would come back again and if it did, what was the miracle which had made it disappear in the first place? Humans need clarification it seems and I was not getting any; at least not just then.

I began to look for answers, discovering books which had been written by others, suggesting a combination of methods which would promote a healing environment and recognized that I had done many of these things. Pure food it seemed was a common requirement and one which I had adhered to, yet my friends had also changed their diets and they had died.

Meditation was definitely recommended and yet, there were those still at the Centre whose disease was not responding to meditation either. Visualization was suggested, especially for children who were experiencing Leukemia and although there had been some successes, there were no guarantees.

The professor had shared some statistics with me which proved that a common factor in those who managed to stay in remission for varying periods of time, hinged on a phenomenon known in the medical profession as the 'healing crisis point'. This apparently was an emotional stage reached by patients where they let go of all expectations relating to the outcome of their disease: that is they didn't care if they lived or died and were peaceful with either outcome.

Interestingly, I had experienced this particular phenomena. In meditation one day as I sat in the stillness I had a sudden thought that despite my desire for the contrary, I might indeed *die*. Strangely, as that thought permeated my consciousness I was quite peaceful with the outcome. Then another thought arose that I might *live*. I waited but still there was only peace. The two thoughts rocked back and forth in my mind like a boat rocking gently on the water: *live* or *die*, *live* or *die*, *live* or *die*. Still there was only peace and with that peace I drifted deep into meditation and the welcoming stillness. Could this be the secret, this letting go of all expectations in the face of calamity and the bringing of a calming peace? Could *peace* be the healing agent? I wondered but still had no answers.

Although I was strangely shy to share my news, it had filtered out to my friends at the Centre. One in particular, a young mother with three children and a diagnosis of advanced Breast Cancer wanted to talk to me about it, so I invited her to come for afternoon tea. As I made the preparations, I selected a rose from a bunch my husband had lovingly given me a few days before. My friend was delighted with the rose and its deep red velvety petals furled in a half bud, and took it home with her. Almost three weeks later it was still fresh and my friend rang me to tell me about its remarkable longevity. The power of love it seems can create miracles.

Chapter Eleven

Oh Ye Of Little Faith

Look now at the unworthiness in your

mind, which tells you that you do not deserve

the gift I have come to give.

The Holy Spirit's Interpretation of the New Testament

A Course in Understanding and Acceptance - Regina Dawn Akers

The Oncologist assured me that the tablets had not been responsible for my recovery.

"It was far too late to offer them" he told me. "I could not however just sit by and do nothing".

As the months wore on, in spite of my seemingly 'miraculous' recovery, my doubts began to gnaw at me.

"What if the disease comes back?" became the refrain which would go over and over in my head. Instead of relishing my victory over illness, I was slowly sabotaging myself.

My youngest daughter had decided to take a break from school before University and was staying in Gurumayi's Ashram in Upstate New York. Her older sister had decided to join her for a time and they would ring me occasionally to see how I was going.

"Have you been to the doctor for your regular check-up?" they would ask innocently.

I dreaded this question as, despite being an intelligent woman, due to my growing doubts, I was avoiding having check-ups like the plague. My mind was beginning to convince me that the doctor was going to find a recurrence and I was going into 'ostrich' mode once more.

After several telephone calls, my girls told me that they had been speaking to Gurumayi who pointed out that Cancer was a very 'tricky' disease and I should go to the doctor for a check-up without delay. That was it. I could no longer avoid the obvious and reluctantly made an appointment to go. Yet, as I sat in the waiting room, and despite my fears, I felt strangely detached from those others who waited. I had after all, been well, although there were often vague and mysterious aches and pains which would sometimes frighten me.

After the examination, the doctor asked me to sit and I waited while he wrote on his cards, carefully straightening them and tapping them on the desk; looking at me over his glasses quietly. He then spoke.

"I don't think you need to come and see me again", he said. "The disease has definitely gone. If you have a recurrence, we shall consider it a new illness and treat it accordingly. How do you feel?"

"Quite well" I managed to babble.

It was amazing I could speak at all, I was so thunderstruck. My head was spinning. The disease had *really* gone. I could hardly believe what I was hearing. Three years had passed since that extraordinary day and although my mind had played tricks on me, here was hard evidence that I was free and clear at last. He shook my hand and wished me well.

"Call me if you need to at any time", he smiled as he closed the door behind me.

This is what I needed hear. I was well, not sick as I had imagined. The miracle was complete. It didn't matter how it had happened; it didn't matter whether it was the food, the meditation, the visualization, the determination, the faith, the affirmations, the surrender or a combination of them all.

"Wasn't life wonderful?" I asked myself as I stepped out of the door onto the footpath.

My feet barely seemed to touch the ground. I could literally taste the air. Happiness was physical I discovered and I was breathing it. The words 'well, well, well' buzzed around in my head like bumble bees. Then it struck me: I had failed to be *grateful* for this amazing good fortune. I had been given a *second* chance at life. I felt very strongly that this had all happened for a reason, that there was something special that I was meant to do only, despite my happiness that day, I was at a loss to know what it was. As I began to think about it, I realized that the sky was the limit. *Everything* that I had ever wanted to do was now there again for me on a platter. I was so excited, I was practically trembling with joy and straining to begin.

There was *so* much I wanted to do and try and I plunged right in. The first attempt was Real Estate. My husband and I had always had a passion for houses, taking orphan properties and fixing them up to sell. This time I would approach it from a different perspective and sell the houses to people as an agent, only I would be the kind of agent who provided such wonderful courteous service that *everyone* would benefit. Through an unusual connection, a real estate job fell into my hands almost immediately and I launched in but as the months rolled by, I became disillusioned with the ethics of my fellow professionals.

The next attempt was at the Law which had beckoned me for years and I approached a friend who worked in a Law firm in the city who immediately gave me a junior position but as I began to contemplate how many years I would have to spend studying and weighed up the small financial compensation for those just starting out in the profession (we had a mortgage after all), I reluctantly withdrew once more. In the interim I continued reading spiritual literature which fed my curiosity about how the universe worked and I began to contemplate going back into the teaching profession which had filled my life for many years and now beckoned me in a new and exciting way.

My experience in the garden the day after the meditation had me on the alert for strange and beautiful occurrences and I was not disappointed. One day as I took a class I was teaching into the church for Mass, the sun was shining down through the stained glass windows onto the heads of the children sitting in front of me. Their hair lit up like molten gold and I wondered at the miracle of this everyday phenomena. Tears began to roll down my cheeks as I gazed at this beautiful sight. One child turned around and asked me if I was alright.

"I am just crying for happy" I responded. The child seemed quite satisfied by this answer; children are very wise after all.

One morning in the space between sleeping and waking I had a dream. In the dream I saw the three women who were my friends at the Cancer Centre who had all died. They were standing together arm-in-arm and smiling at me.

"What are you doing here in my dream?" I asked them.

"We have come to say goodbye" they said fading quickly from view.

I wondered about this dream. Obviously the doctor had confirmed that I was now well, but my friends also seemed to be in on the news; how lovely.

Many years have passed since that time and I am still teaching. These days however I teach many things. I have literally read dozens of books on all kinds of subjects and the more I read, the less I feel I know. Beautiful sights still bring tears to my eyes and as my grandchildren came into the world, I was often there ready to hold them as they entered. Miracles abound in my world yet my life is simple, filled with little daily pleasures: a walk, a good meal, a hug, a kiss a sweet face turned to me in love. I often remember the words I heard in the stillness so many years ago when I asked whoever was listening, what life was all about and realize that the wisdom I received was true:

It is all about love …..

Sandra Munro

EPILOGUE

Chapter Twelve

Meditation

Do you not realize that you have within you all wisdom, all knowledge,

all understanding?

You do not have to seek it without,

but it does mean that you have to take the time

to be still and to go deep within to find it.

Opening Doors Within — Eileen Caddy

There will be many who may wonder what kind of meditation I did during my illness and indeed, the kind of meditation I still practice today. I went on to train to be a Meditation Teacher and am delighted to share the fruits of this knowledge with those who would like to engage in this wonderful practice. Through the techniques set out below, the practitioner can learn at his or her own pace to glide easily into the meditative state and as a result, access benefits which not only facilitate healing but enable them to live life in the fullest possible sense.

When I first learned about Meditation through the writings of Dr. Ainslie Mears, I was completely ignorant of the process. I would sit down in my chair with the book open in front of me and follow the instructions to the letter. Not much happened through this method until one day, after I had come home from work and was feeling quite tired, I sat in the chair and probably due to my fatigued state, was able to truly relax into the process.

Just prior to sitting down, I glanced at the clock which told me the hour was six o'clock, closed my eyes and surrendered and in what seemed like a few seconds, opened them once more only to discover that I had been absent for at least an hour. I have no recollection of what transpired in that hour, I only know that I was not asleep as when I opened my eyes; I was fresh, alert and in a peak state.

When people tell me that they don't know how to meditate, I tell them that meditation is the most natural thing in the world and we do it every day. Have you ever sat watching a sunset or the moon rise; or perhaps a flock of birds moving through a pristine blue sky and during those moments, perhaps feel as though you are somehow absent for a second or two? That is meditation. It is simply a holding of focus on a particular object and if the object of your focus is particularly beautiful, you will glide into that stillness even more quickly.

Have you ever been speaking with a friend when a word they utter will trigger a memory within you? In that moment, you might find yourself becoming so embroiled in your own thoughts that you find you have missed part of what your friend was saying. You apologize for this lapse and refocus. A meditation practice is simply a *deliberate* focusing of thought, enabling you to glide into that place of stillness.

It has been said that we are extensions of Source; some might refer to this as God, the Universe, the Creator, Shiva or whatever name you have chosen to give to this aspect of our being. This non-physical part of you is very wise and not only considers you to be perfect but adores you unconditionally. In some traditions this non-physical aspect of who you are, has been called the *Witness* and it is this part which watches your thoughts at every moment of your waking and sleeping day. When you are in meditation, you are once again reunited with the non-physical part of yourself. In this joining, all knowledge is available to you and you will often get answers to questions, or be shown an internal picture which might answer some problem you are experiencing.

Quite early in my experience of meditation, I was asked by the professor to observe my thoughts as they arose in my awareness. If you have ever tried meditation, you will understand this concept. Once you close your eyes and try to shut out the everyday world, thoughts will arise in your mind with increasing intensity. You might even have an urgent thought such as wondering whether you have left the iron on; or perhaps the lights in your car. You might have an irresistible urge to itch, or even cough; anything which will distract you from the process you are trying to engage in at that moment.

These thoughts are presented to you by what is known as the ego, that part of yourself which engages in logical thought, established beliefs and parameters which have been put in place through long conditioning. When we enter this world we are totally connected to our Source and vibrating with unconditional love. We demand and expect our needs to be met immediately and if they are not, quite rightly complain loudly about it. Have you heard a new baby cry recently? We are after all, non-physical beings having a physical experience and we know before we come that we are creators of our world and even in our baby state, know how to do this instinctively.

However, almost as soon as our mother has her first anxious thought about us, a gap between this pristine part of ourselves, which is an extension of Source, and the physical world is created. As time goes on, parents, siblings, teachers, friends and our environment, all leave their impressions on our psyche until we are so lost in these distortions, that we begin to lose touch, for the most part, with the essence of who we truly are, which is perfection and unconditional love; Source energy if you will.

Of course the ego is not the protagonist here. When we came into the world, although we knew that we were extensions of Source energy, we wanted to create an experience which validated a pseudo-separation from that. In order to do this, the ego was created and it does its job extremely well. Any deliberate steps taken by us to re-enter this stream of consciousness, also known as Source; which occurs in meditation, will be very firmly opposed by the ego. After all its role is to keep our feet planted in the 'real' world we have created. How then do we bypass this intervention?

Giving the mind a focus during the entry process is a tried and true method. Maintaining awareness of the breath, repeating a phrase or mantra or watching a burning candle, are all effective methods to help us gain access to this stream of consciousness. When I was learning to meditate with the professor, he selected chanting the Sanskrit phrase **Om Namah Shivaya,** (which you might remember means *I honor the inner Self)*, followed by a repetition of the same mantra silently on the in-breath and then again on the out-breath for a short period of time, as a means of leading us into meditation.

This particular mantra, imbued with the energy of masters who have used it for centuries, is a very powerful way to lead you into meditation. If you do not wish to use a mantra, just focusing on the natural rhythm of your breath (that is noticing when the inhalation and exhalation take place) will also achieve the same result and once you have glided into meditation, if persistent thoughts begin to surface again, just refocus on the mantra with great gentleness.

Chapter Thirteen

Creative Visualisation

A picture is worth a thousand words.

The subconscious mind will bring to pass any picture held in the mind

and backed by faith:

Act as though I am, and I will be.

The Power of the Subconscious Mind — Joseph Murphy

Another technique I employed when I was trying to get well was Creative Visualization. I first learned of this through the book of the same name written by Shakti Gawain, who espoused its benefits more than twenty years ago. With the understanding that we can create anything we wish with the imagination and, through repetitive thought and focus, can manifest it in our reality, I launched in.

In order to explain this more clearly, think of an invention that is in constant use and you will understand how this concept works; somebody had an idea, mulled it over for a long time, became obsessed by it, pictured it in their mind and eventually received the inspiration to put it into practical application and make it a reality. The telephone and the aeroplane are just two examples.

In my case I wanted *wellness* and as that was not my reality at the time, had to devise a way to trick myself into believing that it was. I would lie down and completely relax, then using the powers of my imagination, create a picture of myself in any way I wished. I was not a particularly athletic person, in fact I often avoided physical activity altogether, so I chose a visualization which incorporated this element as I suspected that physical activity would enhance wellness. Of course even if I was well enough in the beginning to include a daily fitness regime into my life, as the disease unfolded, I definitely was not, so creative visualization was a way to include these benefits without actually performing them physically; at least this is what the book suggested.

I later learned that this form of 'imagining' has been used by world famous athletes, musicians and performers of all kinds as a preparation and refining of their skill. There was even a university research project which pitted the attributes of a renowned basketball team against those of its opponents by preparing the first team with only visualization techniques while the other continued to use physical practice. The thought-motivated team won by several points.

There are also many examples of people who assisted themselves to get well using the power of the mind. One case in particular involved a man from the backwoods who went to the doctor and had a diagnosis of Cancer confirmed. The doctor told him that he would need to go to the city where the specialists had amazing new equipment which could help him.

The man duly travelled to the city and visited with the specialist who asked him to sit on the examination table while he placed a thermometer in his ear to take his temperature. He then proceeded filled out some notes on a form and asked the man to return within a couple of weeks. The man returned and after performing some tests, the specialist could find no trace of the disease. When the man was asked what had happened in the interim, he said that he had been 'cured' by the 'amazing new equipment' used by the doctor.

The mind is a very powerful and the medical profession has called such manifestations, the placebo effect. There are numerous examples of how, through a firm belief in a particular outcome, people have created what might otherwise be considered 'miracles'. When we tap into a place which seems to override everyday reality, we access powers which can move mountains. Great masters have been teaching this for centuries. Jesus, the great master of love said:

"For truly I tell you, if you have faith the size of a mustard seed, you will say to this mountain, "Move from here to there," and it will move; and nothing will be impossible for you".

When we are in a place of fear (which a frightening diagnosis can produce), we need intense focus to bypass such an emotion; creative visualization is an excellent facilitator of this process.

Chapter Fourteen

Diet

We are what we think about all day long

and if we are experiencing any form of

discord, scarcity, sickness or failure,

it's because we've planted these seed

thoughts in the fertile soil of our Creative Mind.

Nothing is Too Good to be True - John Randolph Price

There has been so much written about diet lately that I won't begin to enter this dialogue without the expertise which is now prevalent in this field. I will say however that I had a strong belief (a thought which you think over and over again) that as I was trying to get my body back to wellness, feeding it pure, simple, fresh food was probably the way to go.

As chance would have it, I happened to hear about a doctor who had trained in the Bristol Clinic in England, an institute which was then promoting more alternate ways to heal. The doctor, a warm and caring person, responded to my desire to achieve wellness without the intervention of the usual chemicals being used to treat Cancer, by suggesting that one of the ways to go would be to eat free-range chicken and deep sea fish. These she told me, were less likely to contain the additional elements which could slow down the work which my body was trying to perform. Even twenty years ago, chickens were being fed supplements which could hamper health and fish in the coastal environments, contained higher levels of mercury than those recommended for optimum wellness.

I began this way but soon gave up meat and fish altogether and focused on fresh fruits, vegetables and grains. The holistic doctor also suggested a product called 'Green Magma' which looked and tasted like green talcum powder and which was promoted as a dynamo in creating super health. I discovered a book by Norman Walker, a man who eventually lived well into the hundreds, who espoused the benefits of drinking freshly squeezed fruit and vegetable juices. Following these guidelines, I would make carrot, apple and celery juice (among others) and drink it as often as possible. Dr. Walker suggested that this combination was especially good for those experiencing Cancer. Of course these techniques were new at that time and I felt as though I was groping in the dark but groping was better than standing still I felt; so I got on with it.

Its all about Love

Chapter Fifteen

The Now

Your heart sees beyond the illusions ...

for it knows the greater truth that everything

you ever will have has already been given.

The Keys of Joshua — Glenda Green

In the years that have unfolded since my recovery, I have discovered an astonishing secret. When the body is in perfect alignment with Source (the God-part of you), an alignment which can be achieved through focused thought and meditation; there is no illness.

I can hear your clamoring thoughts:

"But what about the moments which lead up to and after meditation, am I ill then?" If you give attention to your *thoughts* about your illness, you will sustain whatever has been created by original thoughts in the first place. When you are in that place of meditation however, you are in a timeless space which the great ones have referred to as the *NOW*. What is even more extraordinary is that they tell us that there is only the *NOW* and it is in this *NOW* that we create our reality.

I want you to allow yourself to give credence to this idea for a moment. We are creators of our own reality through our focused thoughts and intention. If this is so, why then would you deliberately focus on something you *did not* want (such as illness)? I have given several examples of people who focused on a thought with great belief and achieved results which were considered remarkable; perhaps even miraculous at times. If this is how the universe works, why would you even begin to think of *sickness,* when that is the very thing you are trying to get away from?

This is something which I did not know at the time, yet somehow seemed to stumble upon as if by accident. Here is another piece of interesting information. There are no accidents or coincidences. My focused thought to heal myself without medical intervention had engaged a part of my mind which was sending out vibrations to this effect which, in turn, attracted events or 'coincidences' to me which took me further toward my goal. This process was facilitated by my meditation and visualization practice.

There is however a subtle distinction. Any *striving* towards this goal will take you away from it. Isn't that a contradiction in terms? The focusing on the goal must be done in a relaxed and surrendered way; something that is difficult to achieve when you are in a place of fear or intense wanting. The trick is to use the techniques put forward here to flow past these emotions and take you into the place where you can allow the higher part of you, God if you wish to call it that, to take care of matters. Some have referred to it in this way: **Let go and let God.** If you find any mention of God an anathema, you might like to express it another way: **Let go and go with the** *flow.* The words are not important, it is the way you feel when you are expressing them that is important.

You might remember that at a time when nothing seemed to be working for me I became angry and called out into the stillness to whoever was listening: *What is it all about?* The answer **It's all about love** did not make a lot of sense to me at the time but I have since learned that *love* is who we truly are. God, Source, our creator, the universe; is nothing but *love* and if that is who we are, as extensions of *that* which created the universe, then we too, can create anything we wish. We are after all creators of our world and we came here to be and to enjoy the contrasts we experience, in the process.

What if you were to contemplate the idea that illness is just one of the contrasts you came to experience and that, having discovered that you *did not* want it, chose to focus on what you *did want* instead? Wouldn't that be fun? Perhaps you feel that I lack understanding about the seriousness of your predicament, but let me assure you with the greatest love, that these words I have written contain the secret of life.

Many have written books about this 'secret', their authors having carefully researched, experimented and published, only to have the vital details deliberately left out of the manuscript by the publisher. Why are we afraid to know the truth? Can you imagine a life which was deliberately guided in the direction you wish to go with all the joy that this intention will bring to you?

We are not, as some have suspected, adrift in a sea of intentions where we bob about like corks unable to guide our direction. We are an extension of that power which created the universe, love incarnate. When we realize the wonder of this reality and live our lives accordingly; when our chosen time to depart and return to Source rolls around, those whom we have loved and left behind will shout to the heavens.........*Encore!*